4 Changes

Fix Your Eating & Your Life

by

Anne Katherine

Also by Anne Katherine

To Improve Your Life

Boundaries, Where You End and I Begin

Anatomy of a Food Addiction

Where to Draw the Line

When Misery is Company

How to Make Almost Any Diet Work

Lick It! Fix Her Appetite Switch

Boundaries in an Overconnected World

Your Appetite Switch

The Splintered Cross

Fiction

The Yesterday Doctor

4 Changes

Fix Your Eating & Your Life

Anne Katherine

SoulPath Press

Printed in the United States of America

For information, address Anne Katherine, Box 538, Coupeville, WA 98239 , or email compass@whidbey.net.

www.1annekatherine.com

ISBN: 0692806199
ISBN-13: 978-0692806197 (Soulpath Press)

Dedication

To:
Sherry
Who gives everything

The 4-leggeds
Who also make our house a home

Mamaw and Papaw
Who gave me the start that led to all the good in my life

Anne Katherine

Contents

Warning!

.

Anne Katherine

1 Your Battle with Yourself

You think you *want* to overeat?

You think you would *choose* the daily struggle between foods that call to you and your efforts to resist that call?

With 4 changes, you could find relief.

With just 4 changes, you could rearrange your whole relationship with food and with yourself.

And this struggle has affected your relationship with yourself, hasn't it? You get down on yourself. You've lost some self respect. You think less of you. All because of this food and eating thing, right?

With just 4 changes, this could shift. Dramatically.

Imagine—if this whole struggle were magically lifted, how much more peaceful your inner self would be. Imagine putting your attention to what really matters in your life.

What does really matter to you?

- ☐ To share your life with loved ones.
- ☐ To make progress toward the thing you want most to do.
- ☐ To get a good education so you have lots of choices.
- ☐ To have a healthy, resilient body so you can explore_____. What do you want to

explore?

☐ To have a strong body so you can _____.

What do you want so very much to do?

☐ To feel capable of setting a challenging goal and then of taking each step to get there.

Do you think this struggle will resolve on its own? Will this esteem-lowering issue just go away by itself? When you think about it, you realize it won't. It hasn't thus far, and you've been going through this for...how many years?

How much time and energy are eaten by your internal arguments about eating? How much of your focus is sidetracked from what truly matters? Curious?

Research Yourself—The Coin Transfer Method

For 24 hours, wear something with 2 pockets—a vest, jeans, jacket, waist pack. Put a handful of coins in one pocket—this is your Supply pocket. Every time you think about food, argue with yourself about eating, struggle with a craving, think you should go on a diet, are mad at yourself for messing up your diet, eat too much or the wrong things, feel bad about eating, or make a plan to get food you don't think you should eat, transfer 1 coin to the other pocket. This is your Research pocket.

At the end of 24 hours, count the coins you have transferred to your Research pocket. On your phone, iPad, or laptop, start a note or file entitled *Self Research*.[1]

---

[1] Sample charts are at the end of this book and at my website: www.1annekatherine.com

On the first line, insert the date and number of coins transferred. This represents your thoughts about food, eating, or not eating.

Every single thought took you away from something else.

SELF RESEARCH
2 Jan. 41 thoughts about eating

Every thought used energy you could have used to benefit your life.

FAQ

Q. Should I count normal eating or normal food thoughts?

A. What is normal eating? Many of us have lost touch with the definition of normal eating. Normal food thoughts according to whom—*People Magazine*, Dr. Phil, cereal ads, or your mother?

Count *all* thoughts about eating and food. Count all efforts involved in either getting or resisting food.

Q. How do I count a binge?

A. Transfer 1 coin for each 15 minutes of a binge.

If your eating starts with a meal, but doesn't stop after 45 minutes, count every additional 15 minutes of nearly continuous eating.

For example, you start eating dinner at 6:00 and continue eating for a total of 2 hours. Transfer a coin each for 6:45, 7:00, 7:15, 7:30, and 7:45, making a total of 5 coins.

If you find yourself trying to cheat this system, by stopping eating after 44 minutes, waiting 15 minutes, and then eating more, count every effort to cheat the system.

The exception: an elegant meal that lasts two hours because you are savoring each course and conversing with a companion. This is not a binge and doesn't require coin transfer.

You are paying attention in a new way and you will soon discriminate between a savored meal and craving-induced eating. Do not count savored meals. Most of us binge eat when we are alone. (And most of us do not savor even our favorite foods on a binge.)

My question for you:

To whom are you responsible for the way you live your life?

- ☐ Facebook Friends
- ☐ Social Media Public
- ☐ Mom
- ☐ Dad
- ☐ Yourself
- ☐ _____

I hope you picked yourself, which is why you should be honest with yourself as you do this research. Accuracy will give you a way to see the big difference these 4 changes make.

You are beginning a transition to a new normal.

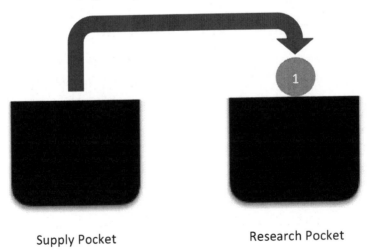

Supply Pocket   Research Pocket

Getting More Conscious

How many times did I pretend to not notice that I was organizing myself for a binge? These thoughts can be so slippery that we can be planning a binge while telling someone who trusts us that we are just going to the library.

Any of the following is a reason to transfer a coin:

Thoughts	Feelings	Actions
Gotta get candy.	Gotta have sugar.	Making a plan to eat food that is bad for you.
Boss has dish on desk. Walk by. Grab some.	Desperate.	Making a plan to get food that can harm you.
Eating is bad. I'm bad.	Need comfort.	Making a plan to hide food or eating.
Leftover dessert in fridge.	Empty.	Gathering sweets surreptitiously.
I shouldn't eat.	Need filling.	Concocting schemes that hide what you are really doing.
I'm skipping lunch.	Lonely. Need relief.	Lying about eating.
I'm going to that drive thru.	Longing. Gotta eat.	Hiding food.
I'll just have 1 more.	Overwhelmed.	Hiding eating.
I'll just have 2 more.	Can't stop.	Concealing your portion.
I'll just have 1 more.	Driven to eat.	Hiding a sweet under lettuce.
I'm fat.	Need food fix.	Inhaling food.
I'll start the Wild diet.	Want it.	Shoving food in.
The bakery is open.	Gotta stop this feeling.	Searching for dropped crumb while driving.
I'll drive myself then I can go to dessert store.	Gotta be less aware.	Planning to restrict your eating.
Sneak into kitchen.	Need to numb feelings.	Bingeing
Take bits so no one notices.	Craving	Arguing with yourself about eating.
	I'm all alone.	Overeating.

2 They Make You Eat

Do you *want* to overeat?

Of course not. Most of the overeaters I know, including my young self, longed to be a normal eater. We absolutely, positively could not fathom how someone could eat half a cookie or leave part of a piece of pie on the plate. But we sure wanted to be that person.

You eat because chemicals in your body push you to eat. You overeat for the same reason. You can prove this to yourself.

Think back to the time you were sick and didn't feel like eating. How about the time someone offered you boiled liver or cod marinated in lye. Think about this morning.

Did you feel like eating when you woke up?

Why *are* you desperate to eat a giant whatever on your way home from work and completely uninterested in eating when you wake up?

Because overnight your body chemicals changed.

Guess what? You can change them yourself.

And *that* will change your eating.

3 You are Driven

That's right, chemicals in your body drive you to think about food and to feel desperate about eating. Other chemicals *should* tell you when to stop eating.

If your eating is out of balance, it proves that your chemicals are out of balance.

The only lasting solution to this problem is to fix your chemical balance. Two of the chemicals are easy to change—if you will commit yourself to keeping them changed.

In my 40 years working with, mostly, women with appetite disorder, they found it hard to sustain easy changes. What made it hard? Getting distracted.

Women are easily distracted from taking care of themselves.

You'd almost think they were still being taught that other people are more important. Or that following the rules is more important. Or that washing dishes is more important. Or recycling is more important. Or picking the speck of lint off that sweater.

Of course many of these things matter, but nothing matters more than keeping yourself healthy. Your own health enables you to do every other important thing.

And beating up on yourself for a bossy chemical imbalance is not healthy.

How hard is it to make these four changes?

You can make the first two changes easily.

The third change seems hard at first, then gets easier. The fourth change is really hard at first, gets easier after 3 weeks, and becomes a way of life.

And **you have to keep doing** the things that make your body chemicals change.

It's not like setting a thermostat. It's much more like charging your phone. You have to do it every day.

Still, it takes maybe 15 minutes of attention every day to sustain the changes. Perhaps it takes another hour per week to make sure you have what you need.

How many coins did you transfer between pockets on your first self-research project? How many food struggle thoughts did you endure? How many minutes are represented by those coins?

Which is more economical: 15 minutes a day or _____ minutes of struggling and thinking bad thoughts about yourself?

4 Tummy vs. Brain

Do you have 3 pockets?

Here's one more thing to study before the first change—the difference between hunger and appetite.

Hunger is a sensation, mostly felt in the tummy. Appetite is a drive, an urge. Both are chemically mediated, but hunger is usually not the issue that makes you overeat—unless you get too hungry.

Can you remember a time that you were hungry but had no appetite? Even though you knew you needed food, you didn't *want* food.

How about appetite without hunger? How recently did you eat even though you weren't hungry? And you knew you weren't hungry. You might even have been full and you still couldn't stop.

These examples illustrate that there's a difference between the two, between the processes involving appetite vs. those that involve hunger.

Hunger is resolved by eating.

Appetite, however, is resolved by a decrease in appetite-causing chemicals and an increase in satiety chemicals.

Satiety is the opposite of appetite. It is caused by stop-eating body chemicals. It means the brain is satisfied with your nutritional intake.

Changes 1, 3, and 4 will decrease powerful appetite-causing chemicals.

Changes 1 and 2 will increase satiety chemicals.

But first, your job is to get smarter about the difference between your own hunger signals and your appetite signals.

Observing Hunger versus Appetite

You'll need 3 pockets.

In one supply pocket put one type of coin, for example, pennies. In another supply pocket put a different type of coin, for example, nickels. Designate one coin as hunger and the other coin as appetite.

For the next 24 hours, whenever you feel hungry, transfer the hunger coin to the Research pocket, your third pocket. Whenever you are feeling pushed to eat, fixated on a particular food, craving a food, planning a strategy for eating, being distracted by the thought of eating, eating due to a craving, or binge eating (eating that lasts more than 45 minutes or cheating the system), transfer an appetite coin to the Research pocket.

At the end of 24 hours, count the two types of coins.

Record the totals on your Self Research chart. [2]

SELF RESEARCH
2 Jan. 41 thoughts about eating
3 Jan. 6 hunger coins. 27 appetite coins.

---

[2] You can find sample charts at the end of this book and at www.1annekatherine.com.

What did you learn about the difference between hunger and appetite? If you feel like it, tell what you learned to a friend.

```
┌─────────────────────────────┐
│  Nosh Partake Yes           │
└─────────────────────────────┘
```

5 NPY

NPY, neuro-peptide Y, is a major appetite stimulator.
It's a body chemical, a protein fragment called a peptide.

Certain actions cause NPY to increase.

When it increases, you are **driven** to eat. **DRIVEN**. It is
50 times more powerful than most other appetite stimulating
chemicals. It's one of the appetite chemicals that makes it hard for
you to stop eating once you start.

Do you think you can defy body chemistry?

Can you make yourself stay awake for a week (without
getting bonkers)? Can you hold your breath for 20 minutes? How
about stopping your period once it starts to flow? Can you make
your hair grow faster?

As mental and virtual as we've become, the body is still
running things. In fact, the body is so insistent, that if you skip or
delay meals, it releases NPY so that when you do start eating,
you'll find it harder to stop.

Clients have told me at least 5000 times that they have no
trouble missing breakfast and even lunch, but then, after work,

they can't keep themselves from eating non-stop for hours.

The reality is this:

> **The** longer you delay eating, the more NPY builds up, **and when you do eat, it will control you.**

People delay eating for lots of reasons, but underneath the reasons may be a persistent attitude that goes something like this: "I'm bad when I eat. I'm good when I don't eat."

Do you think that way too? Do you think not eating is a virtue?

Food is one of the main necessities for survival.

Survival is success.

Since you are getting more conscious, notice how many ways that attitude is expressed around you. Notice comments like, "I know I shouldn't eat this, but..."

Notice bargaining for food, as if you have to sacrifice or earn the right to eat. For example, "I missed breakfast and lunch and rescued 30 kids from stampeding horses. I deserve this sugar bar."

Our culture surrounds us with mixed messages, half urging us to buy that fluffy new carb from Mama Dough, the other half hawking the Only Diet that Works or the machine that takes off a pound a minute.

Do you believe, deep down, you shouldn't eat? If so, know that by delaying meals, you are setting yourself up to have a BIG appetite.

Change 1 has two parts. Here's the first half:

Change 1a—Manage NPY. Eat 3 meals a day.

This change is to bring you up to normal. It is normal to eat three meals a day. If you've been skipping meals out of a mistaken belief that eating is bad, it will be surprisingly uncomfortable to make sure you have three daily meals.

> **I**
> **D**
> **O**
> **N'**
> **T**
>
> **E**
> **A**
> **T**
>
> **B**
> **R**
> **E**
> **A**
> **K**
> **F**
> **A**
> **S**
> **T**

1. It doesn't have to be a big meal.

2. It *does* have to include protein.

Breakfast can be 2 cheese sticks or a half cup of cottage cheese or a cup of soy milk. It can be a peanut butter sandwich, a handful of almonds, cheese toast, yogurt, a hard-boiled egg, a slice of meat.

Despite convincing statistics that skipping breakfast is a bugaboo, an alarming percentage do it. People have reasons, but few hold water.

Don't have the time. Slide cheese sticks into your pocket.

Don't want to go to the trouble. Carry a bag of almonds in your purse or pack.

Can't think about this in the morning. Think about it the night before. I mean, really, it takes 10 seconds to throw some trail mix into a baggie and put it in your pack.

Don't want to cook. Ditto the above.

———

Like I said, most excuses don't hold water. But this whole argument is showing you something.

It's showing you that you do have a working satiety chemical. It's just working at the wrong time.

Want to check your progress?

After you've succeeded in having 3 meals each day, for at least 3 days in a row, fill up your supply pocket with coins. For 24 hours, transfer one coin each time you feel pushed to eat, get obsessed with a certain food, or notice that push/pull attitude—eating is wrong, not eating is right—or any of the other thoughts, feelings, or actions that circle this issue for you.

After 24 hours, count the coins in your Research pocket. Record that total in your chart.

SELF RESEARCH
2 Jan. 41 coins
7 Jan. Change 1a. 31 coins.

Here are three more reasons to make Change 1 and decrease your NPY:

- NPY promotes fat buildup.
- NPY promotes insulin resistance.
- NPY reduces the production of leptin—the brain chemical that tells you to stop eating fatty foods.

You definitely want to stop your body from over-producing NPY.

The remedy? Change 1a.

Do you believe that not eating is a virtue or that you are being good when you don't eat?

Can you go back in time to your early life before you thought skinny celebrities on TV or YouTube represented model womanhood or to a boyhood in which you freely ripped off your shirt without concern about your belly being judged?

Believe it or not, when you were really young, you ate happily. You felt okay about wanting food.

Notice any negative thoughts you have about regular meals, and reframe them to yourself. For example, *food is necessary. I eat to survive.*

FAQ

Q. Should I try to discriminate between hunger and appetite in my Self Research?

A. No. Don't side-track yourself with perfection. Count all indicators that show thoughts, feelings, or actions that have to do with eating, not eating, or fighting with yourself about eating. Keep it simple. You can refer to the list on page 5, or you can develop your own list of indicators.

6 PYY-Please

PYY says, "Step away from the fridge, Ma'am. Put the bag down slowly. Exit the kitchen."

PYY, peptide YY, is the stop eating body chemical. If NPY says *Yes*, PYY says *No*, at least to 2nd helpings.

PYY is a powerful satiety chemical and every time you skip a meal, it decreases. Over time, it can be quite delayed in action. Some think that PYY delay is genetically determined as well, and that one cause of obesity in families is due to a delay in PYY activation.

The arguments don't really matter because you can build up your PYY.

And you want to do this. PYY can also motivate you to exercise and can raise your metabolism.

Change the chemical and the body changes.

It makes sense that if the body thinks you are starving, it's not gonna produce a chemical that stops you from eating, encourages you to move, or that burns calories.

See how all this works? You have to convince your body you aren't starving. You do this by adding two small protein snacks a day.

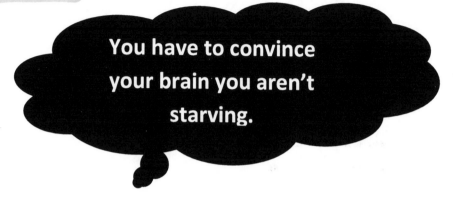

You have to convince your brain you aren't starving.

If you are just now getting used to 3 meals a day, you might have to wait a week or so before tackling the rest of change 1. Up to you.

The entire Change 1 is this: Eat 5 meals or snacks each day, making sure you have some protein each time.

The order isn't too important. You can have a snack, then breakfast, then lunch, a snack, and dinner. You can have dinner for breakfast and breakfast for dinner. It doesn't matter what you call it.

Just have some protein 5 times a day, every two or three hours.

Protein builds up PYY and increases metabolism.

Want to check your progress? After you've implemented Change 1 for at least 5 days in a row, fill your supply pocket with coins. You know the drill. Transfer a coin each time you have an indicator (page 5). After 24 hours, count the coins. Record the totals in your chart.

> **SELF RESEARCH**
> 2 Jan.   41 coins
> 7 Jan. Change 1a. 31 coins.
> 12 Jan. Change 1. 19 coins.

PYY is the answer to NPY.

PYY reduces insulin resistance.

PYY stops appetite.

PYY stops eating.

7 Trypping Out

Serotonin is a major satiety chemical. It also reduces stress, slows eating, spreads calm, decreases depression, increases a sense of well-being. For some, it even reduces irritability and crankiness. It's pretty great.

It's a neurochemical that is manufactured inside the body. You can't take it as a pill. You can't eat it.

You can eat the chemical that gets it made. Tryptophan is the essential ingredient that is converted to serotonin.

Most people are walking around with a serotonin deficit, because whenever we are in pain or stressed—like all the time— serotonin gets used up. And if our tryptophan intake isn't matching our serotonin consumption, we get a quart low pretty quickly.

This is easily fixed. Change 2. Keep serotonin supplied. Eat tryptophan-effective foods.

(You may have noticed that changes 1 and 2 involve eating more of something. This isn't looking like a diet, is it? In fact, the concept of dieting works against appetite management.)

Serotonin works throughout the body and also in the brain. Its effectiveness in the brain depends on tryptophan crossing through a barrier that protects the brain from chemicals that would be too concentrated for its tender cells (the blood-brain barrier).

You succeed at change 2 by eating foods that send tryptophan into the brain. The best sources are turkey and milk. Sesame seeds run a semi-distant third.

Lactose intolerant? Eat turkey. If you are a vegetarian, drink milk. If you are a vegan, sesame seeds and tahini are your friends. If you are a lactose intolerant vegetarian, ditto.

Dose is important. On an ordinary week, you need the equivalent of 4 ounces of turkey at least 3 times during the week. Four measures, four times a week, is better. That's 4 X 4: 4 measures, 4 days, each week.

If you are in pain or stressed, your need increases. When you travel, your routine is interrupted, you have a sick kid or spouse, are facing a test or deadline, you need more tryptophan enhancing foods.

The following chart gives equivalencies:

Food	1 Measure	4 Measures	Preferred Weekly
Turkey-White meat	1 ounce	4 ounces	16 Ounces (1 pound)
Turkey-Dark meat	1.5 oz.	6 oz.	24 oz. (1.5 lb.)
Turkey slices-packaged	2 oz.	8 oz.	32 oz. (2 pounds)
Milk-whole	4.5 oz.	18 oz. or 2.25 cups	72 oz. (9 cups or 2¼ quarts)

Milk-Low fat	7 oz.	28 oz. or 3.5 C	112 oz. (14 cups or 3½ quarts)
Yogurt	11 oz.	44 oz. or 5.5 C	176 oz. (22 cups or 11 pints)
Sesame Seeds	1 oz.	4 oz.	16 oz. (1 pound)
Tahini	1 oz.	4 oz.	16 oz.
Sesame Oil	1 oz.	4 oz.	16 oz.
Soy Milk	5.5 oz.	23 oz. (almost 3 cups)	92 oz. (11.5 cups or nearly 3 quarts)
Mozzarella	Half oz. plus	2 1/3 oz.	9.33 oz.
Parmesan	2/3 oz.	2.5 oz.	10 oz.
Ricotta	2.5 oz.	10 oz.	40 oz (2.5 pounds)
Cottage cheese	2.5 oz.	10 oz.	40 oz (2.5 pounds)
Pumpkin Seeds	1 oz.	4 oz.	16 oz.

Is chicken as good as turkey? No. Don't know why.

Are pumpkin seeds as effective as sesame seeds? No. Don't know why.

Is cheddar as good as ricotta? No. Somehow the processing kills an enzyme that tryptophan uses in the brain. At least that's my theory.

My theory is that a particular enzyme in certain foods supports the effectiveness of tryptophan in the brain. I can't tell you why, but the foods in the chart work better than other foods with just as much tryptophan.

Once tryptophan is in the blood stream, it still has to cross into the brain. Carbohydrates are the mechanism that facilitate that crossing. The absolutely perfect meal is the traditional

American Thanksgiving meal—high in both tryptophan and carbs. No wonder people get sleepy.

You don't have to orchestrate the brain crossover. If you are careful to keep tryptophan routinely supplied to the bloodstream, it will transfer into the brain with your other eating.

However, if you need a direct hit—for example, are under serious stress or need sleep—have a glass of warm milk with a teaspoon of honey and, about 20 minutes later, a biscuit, rice, or oatmeal. (Those old wives knew a thing or two.)

Change 2. Make sure you have 4 measures of foods in the chart at least 3 days a week (the minimum). Even better, have 4 measures of those foods 4 days per week (preferred). You can mix food sources. You can spread them out over the week.

If it's been awhile since you've had any of these foods, eat 4 measures every day for a week, then maintain a routine of four measures a day, 3 or 4 days each week.

Will pills do? No!

And if you are on *antidepressants*, you must **not** get your tryptophan from pills.

If you are *pregnant*, you must **not** get your tryptophan from pills.

Eat it!

> **If you are on antidepressants,**
> **you must not get your tryptophan from pills.**
>
> **If you are pregnant, you must not get your tryptophan from pills.**

How can you tell you are not eating enough tryptophan? Your appetite will increase.

If your appetite increases, you need to increase your intake. After awhile, you'll begin to learn what your optimal dose is.

Want to watch your progress? After a week of the preferred measure of tryptophan, research yourself.

```
SELF RESEARCH
2 Jan.  41 coins
7 Jan. Change 1a. 31 coins.
12 Jan. Change 1. 23 coins.
19 Jan. Change 2. 19 coins.
```

Hoarding

Serotonin, in animals, affects perception of food supply. With insufficient serotonin, food looks scarce.

Some of us like to shop. Some of us hoard. Could it be that low serotonin makes us concerned about not having enough?

Wouldn't it be interesting if your desire to hang on to or acquire things decreased as you maintained tryptophan levels? Might be worth noticing.

Tryptophan promotes satiety.

Tryptophan helps sleep, which also promotes appetite regulation and healing.

Tryptophan reduces stress.

Be sure to keep change 1 going after you add change 2.

To form a habit, research shows you have to sustain a practice for 21 days, (so the brain can build new connections). Then the change becomes routine.

Anne Katherine

Are you willing to sustain Changes 1 and 2 for 21 days?

8 Spacing

The body fixes itself with amazing speed if you give it the help it needs.

How long have you had a problem with an overactive appetite? 5 years? 20 years? Since you were 10?

Then it's pretty amazing that after about a month, your appetite will begin to right itself, with all 4 changes.

Not saying you have to be perfect at all 4 changes right away. Not saying you have to be graceful or good at it at the beginning.

If you were sleep deprived for a year and started to get almost enough sleep for one night, the body would make use of that.

Your body will notice that the need for NPY has gone down. It will notice that you aren't starving and start producing PYY. It will use tryptophan instantly—like a drooping petunia when the ground is finally watered.

How quickly will your body regain a proper balance of appetite and satiety chemicals? Pretty darn fast considering how long it's not been helped.

You are helping it now, instead of fighting it.

Consider. To the body, many diets send a message of starvation. The body will always make drastic adjustments to keep you alive during famine. When you used a diet to get rid of weight, particularly an extreme diet, your body hunkered to down to save you from starving. You were fighting each other.

The body always wins, even if winning the battle loses the war.

(It wins by saving you from famine, but all of the body's defenses against starvation cause you to store weight. In the long run, that weight hurts you, making you vulnerable to diabetes and other problems. But the body is concerned about today's fight, not some fight in the future.)

Want to get rid of weight? Be persistent about maintaining the 4 changes. Gradually all sorts of systems kick in, like—in about 6 months—a desire to exercise.

How should you space the changes?

Depends on whether it is important to you to see the degree of difference each change makes, or if you've been down on yourself, or if you tend to act on impulse.

If you like to think things through and you want to have verifiable results, give each Change one week before starting the next one.

Do Self Research just before starting each new Change, and you'll get to see how each change lowers your appetite. This will prove to you that this whole overeating problem was a chemical issue all along and never meant you were weak or lacking in discipline.

But you may prefer to ride the wave. While your motivation is hot, you may want to get the whole show going.

That's okay. Particularly if that's worked for you in the past.

What if that doesn't work for you, not really. What if diving deep sets you up to get overwhelmed and throw out the entire thing?

Moderation?

You can start over, giving each change more time, or you can find some compromise between overwhelming yourself and riding the wave.

For example, start Changes 1 and 2, and then proceed to Change 3 after a week of getting used to the new eating structure.

Or start Changes 1 and 2, wait 3 days before adding Change 3 and then wait another week before adding Change 4. You know your pattern. You can orchestrate these changes to take advantage of what you already know about yourself.

Those of us who have battled our appetite's tyranny for a long time may want to leap aboard while at the same time carrying a deep belief that nothing will ever work. We have already given up on a fundamental level. We think we'll be running around this wheel forever, like a crazed guinea pig.

If this is your story, do those coin counting tests. You'll get external validation that each Change you make works. This will help you change more than your appetite. You will also have a reason to change your beliefs about yourself.

9 Eating to Stop Feelings

password

Stress increases NPY. Stress uses up (serotonin.) You are already helping yourself with your first 2 changes.

Now we'll look at the other major reason for eating—to feel better, or, at least, to block (feelings.)

I had a vivid demonstration of this use of food some decades ago, after a day with my mother.

By then, I'd been in recovery from food addiction for many years. I was an expert on food addiction and had developed programs for recovery. But after a day with my mother, I felt a bottomless emptiness.

I ate until I was hurting. My gut was so distended I was in physical distress, but I still felt empty. I crammed food into my mouth. I couldn't get enough. I couldn't get enough.

I finally remembered to call a close friend. I told her what I was experiencing. Her kindness and empathy gave me enough comfort to stop eating.

If you have a good friend, someone you can talk to when you are upset, this is the best solution. And sometimes we don't have a friend like that. And sometimes we don't remember to reach out. And sometimes that's the hardest time to reach out.

So another important tool is to be able to make room for feelings.

Until we learn to do this, food is the fastest, best comfort. And it takes a lot of practice for anything else to be as good. But if you are willing to keep practicing, and if you are willing to keep giving this tool a shot, it eventually can make the huge, lasting, transformative difference, not just to your eating, but to your life.

Change 3. Make Room. Make room for what you are feeling.

I know this isn't as simple as it sounds, at least not at first. (We'll practice this in little steps in a moment.)

If you're like I used to be, you've been avoiding feelings for years. You don't even know what you're not feeling. You may not experience joy all that much either. When we get into the habit of turning away from our internal experience, we can miss happiness as well as misery.

We can also be selective avoiders. Men may avoid sadness by substituting anger or rage. Most common among women is to avoid anger and substitute either self blame or sadness.

Perpetual avoidance of true anger creates depression, not necessarily chemical depression, but the lose-all-energy, can't get-things-done or compulsive-overdoer, kind of depression. Well, that involves chemicals too and the two kinds of depression can enhance each other, but the bottom line is this: avoiding true anger (different from rage or outrage) can cause or enhance depression.

Those of us who were hurt by something as children and

who weren't taught how to contain feelings are most vulnerable to avoiding feelings.

Some of us were actively taught to shut feelings off: "I'll give you something to cry about."

We learned to survive by avoiding feelings that seemed lethal—either too much to bear or too dangerous to reveal to hair-trigger parents.

We survived. We were successful.

But now, avoidance is shutting out a part of your life experience. You are missing a primary aspect of human life.

You could also be missing your very best guidance—your own inner wisdom. Avoidance gets in the way of your wise inner voice.

Inside of you is deep knowledge about which choices are best for you. You have a purpose. You have a unique path. All of this is hidden in the vault created by avoidance.

Until you unlock that vault, you are prone to going the wrong direction, using maps provided by your family, your culture, your gang, your workplace, YouTube, media, or advertisers. The map may be a good one, but it isn't yours.

Your life matters. You are here for a reason. Your job is to discover that reason. You can find it, if you learn how to counteract a tendency toward avoidance.

Most of the following steps take less than 5 minutes. Are you willing to experiment for just 5 minutes to see if discovering more about yourself can make a radical improvement in your quality of life?

Section 1. Preparation for Making Room

We generally don't make steam from ice. We melt the ice to create water, and then we heat the water to make steam.

Similarly, we prepare ourselves to Make Room. Section 1 gives you tools that prepare you for Section 2--Making Room.

Your first time through, practice the prep steps in order. Start with Prep Step 1, then continue with Prep Step 2, either at that same sitting or at a later time.

Even when you are familiar with the steps listed in Section 2, Making Room, do at least one prep step any time you begin to Make Room.[3]

Do not practice any of these steps while driving or operating machinery.

Use good judgment if you are responsible for the care of someone else.

All steps in both sections are most effective if you do the following:

- Go to a private place where you can shut the door and be alone, if possible.
- Turn off videos, TV, and music. Turn off the ring tone on the phone.
- Sit in an upright chair, not a couch or easy chair, so that your spine can be in alignment. A desk chair can work well.
- Sit with both feet flat on the floor.

---

[3] Would you prefer to hear, rather than read, these steps? Go to www.1annekatherine.com.

Prep Step 1. Pause.

1. Right now, pause, for 2 minutes.
2. Notice what sounds you can hear.
3. Notice the colors around you.
4. Become aware of touches on your skin—from fabric, your chair, temperature.
5. Take two slow breaths.
6. Notice what is happening inside your body right now.

Notice Yourself

How did that go?

Was it manageable? How do you feel right now?

You can, if you think it would be helpful, jot down some notes about what you learned from this. Or you can tell a friend.

You may go on to the next step now, or you can practice this step again tomorrow and/or wait a few days before moving forward.

You may follow any of these steps with the Comfort Step, later in this chapter.

Prep Step 2. Look Inside

Look inside yourself for 4 minutes.

1. Pause.
2. Become aware of your skin. Notice where your skin is warm and where it is cool. Hold both the awareness of cold and the awareness of warm at the same time.
3. Let your awareness sink through your skin to your muscles. Notice what muscles are tense and which

ones are relaxed. Which muscles are sore and which ones comfortable. Become aware of your entire musculature at once.

4. Let your awareness sink through your muscles to your bones. How are your bones feeling? Are they at rest? Are they strong? Do any of your bones ache? Are your bones tired?

5. Simply notice. Let your bones be as they are. What is it like to not push your bones to feel differently than they actually feel?

6. If you want, let your awareness now travel along your nerve pathways. Trace a nerve from your head to your fingers, from your toe to your neck. They are like lightning fast public transportation.

7. Become aware of your heart. Focus all your attention on your heart area.

8. Notice what is happening in your body right now?

Notice Yourself

How did that go?

Was it manageable? How do you feel right now?

You can, if you think it would be helpful, jot down some notes about what you learned from this. Or you can tell a friend.

You may go on to the next step now, or you can practice this step again tomorrow and/or wait a few days before moving forward.

Prep Step 3. Center

Sink into your center for 5 minutes.

1. Pause.
2. Place your feet flat on the floor.
3. Notice the position of your body. Is it out of alignment?
4. Align your spine, so that your right and left sides are balanced.
5. Check that you are balanced from front to back.
6. Notice your hands. Allow them to relax.
7. Notice your shoulders. Let them become heavier.
8. Notice your breathing.
9. Breathe, slowly, and notice the sensation of the breath traveling through your nostrils, down your throat, into your chest, into your lungs.
10. Exhale slowly and notice the sensation of the breath traveling up through your lungs, up your throat, through your nostrils, to the outside.
11. Again, inhale slowly. Notice the passage of the breath from outside of you all the way to your diaphragm. Feel the expansion of your diaphragm. Feel the filling.
12. Exhale slowly. Feel your diaphragm pushing air out, all the way to the outside of your body. Feel the release.
13. On your next inhale, focus on the filling.
14. On your next exhale, focus on the release.
15. With your next breath, breathe all the way to your toes.
16. As the breath releases, stay deep.
17. Sink into your very center.
18. What is it like?

19. Is it still? A stillness.

20. Is it quiet?

21. If not, what is it like?

22. Simply notice.

23. Stay there as long as you like.

24. Notice what is happening in your body right now?

Notice Yourself

How did that go?

Was it manageable? How do you feel right now?

You can, if you think it would be helpful, jot down some notes about what you learned from this. Or you can tell a friend.

You may go on to the next step now, or you can practice this step again tomorrow and/or wait a few days before moving forward.

Extra Credit Prep Step 4. Playing with Stillness

This step is optional, but it is an interesting alternative to eating to mask feelings.

1. Pause. Follow each sub-step of Prep Step 1.

2. Look inside. Sink down through your layers.

3. Focus on your breathing, on the rhythm of filling and releasing.

4. Center. Find stillness.

5. Inside your center, sense your own soul. Notice your soul. How big is it? Does it have color?

6. Sense the energy of the planet.

7. Sense the flow of energy between you and the planet.

8. Sense the energy of the universe.

9. Sense your connection with all that is.

Notice Yourself

How did that go?

Was it manageable? How do you feel right now?

You can, if you think it would be helpful, jot down some notes about what you learned from this. Or you can tell a friend.

Section 2. Making Room

After preparing yourself with at least one prep step, use one of the following steps to actually Make Room.

The first time you do this, start with Step 1, then wait at least one day before moving on to Step 2. Advance through the steps as more difficult feelings present themselves, taking some recovery time in between steps.

Once you've practiced on a hard feeling, use any of the steps whenever you become aware that some feeling inside you is being repressed, stifled, or avoided.

At any point, it is okay to ask for help, either from a trusted friend who knows how to feel her own feelings, or from a professional who can guide you through the process.

Do not ask for help from someone you don't trust, someone who has hurt you when you've revealed yourself in the past, or someone who will use what you say against you.

At the end of the book is a list of resources you can use to find fellow self-explorers.

Step 1. Make Room for an easy feeling.

1. At an ordinary time, use one of the Prep Steps in

Section 1.

2. Notice a feeling you are having right now.

3. Simply notice that feeling.

4. Imagine giving that feeling all the space it wants.

5. Now give it more space.

6. Give it more space.

7. Notice what happens.

8. What does the feeling do?

9. Keep watching the feeling.

10. The feeling may turn into a different feeling.

11. It may offer you an insight.

12. It may—poof--disappear.

13. Notice what is happening in your body right now?

Notice Yourself

How did that go?

Was it manageable? How do you feel right now?

You can, if you think it would be helpful, jot down some notes about what you learned from this. Or you can tell a friend.

You may want to finish with The Comfort Step.

Step 2. Make Room for a slightly more challenging feeling.

1. Use one of the Prep Steps in Section 1.

2. Notice a feeling you are having right now, a feeling you would ordinarily shy away from.

3. Simply notice that feeling.

4. Imagine giving that feeling all the space it wants.

5. Now give it more space.

6. Give it more space.

7. Notice what happens.

8. What does the feeling do?

9. Keep watching the feeling.

10. The feeling may turn into a different feeling.

11. It may offer you an insight or wisdom.

12. It may—poof—disappear.

13. Notice what is happening in your body right now?

Notice Yourself

How did that go?

Was it manageable? How do you feel right now?

You can, if you think it would be helpful, jot down some notes about what you learned from this. Or you can tell a friend.

You may want to finish with The Comfort Step.

Step 3. Make Room for a hard feeling.

1. Use one of the Prep Steps in Section 1.

2. Notice a feeling you are having right now, a feeling that is usually difficult for you to feel.

3. Simply notice that feeling.

4. Imagine giving that feeling all the space it wants.

5. Now give it more space.

6. Give it more space.

7. Notice what happens.

8. What does the feeling do?

9. Keep watching the feeling.

10. The feeling may turn into a different feeling.

11. It may offer you an insight. You may suddenly realize something.

12. It may—poof—disappear.

13. Notice what is happening in your body right now?

Notice Yourself

How did that go?

Was it manageable? How do you feel right now?

You can, if you think it would be helpful, jot down some notes about what you learned from this. Or you can tell a friend.

Anger vs. Sadness

Most of us who have repressed feelings have too little anger and tend to hold back. It takes time to learn how to be safe and to trust that we can be in charge of ourselves even when we're angry.

For some of us, though, anger is our go-to feeling. If you are in this sub-group, you may have more difficulty feeling sorrow or sadness. Your job then, is to bring yourself back to a sad feeling rather than let it be converted to anger. Use the Make Room steps, and when you come to the end of those steps, add one more step: The Comfort Step.

The Comfort Step

After any Make Room process, you can end with the Comfort Step.

1. Put your arms around yourself.

2. Tell yourself you are worthy of being loved. You are good. You are dear.

3. Feel loving arms around you.

4. Breathe in love for yourself.

5. Imagine that you are your own loving grandmother, even if you didn't have a loving grandmother, or think of someone who was a kind grandmother of a friend or in a movie. Imagine that she is holding you with all the love in the world.

6. Soak up love.

7. Soak up love.

Advanced Application

What if it's a *really* hard feeling? Making Room works no matter what the feeling is. It's an all-purpose tool.

There is an advanced application. This involves allowing the feeling some physical expression, but there are rules.

Before you practice the next process, read the rules:

Rules for Physical Expression of Feelings

1. You aren't allowed to hurt yourself.

2. You aren't allowed to hurt anyone else.

3. You aren't allowed to destroy anything that matters.

4. You can throw ice, outside, at a strong wall.

5. You can yell (if all children are out of hearing range. They have good hearing.)

6. You can say any metaphor, but if it is graphic, either say it so no one can hear or prepare a listener in advance, like before you even get into this.

7. You can beat on a fat pillow.

8. If at any point, it feels like too much feeling, or if you start thinking about hurting yourself or someone else,

cool yourself down. Distract yourself with TV or music. Go for a walk. Call a friend. Go to a 12 step meeting. Call a pastor, Help Line, or therapist. Don't try this again until you have an effective person to help you.

9. Go back to the Comfort Step.

Step 4. Allow boundaried expression of a feeling.

Follow the rules.

1. Use one of the Prep Steps in Section 1.
2. Notice a feeling you are having right now.
3. Simply notice that feeling.
4. Imagine giving that feeling all the space it wants.
5. Now give it more space.
6. Give it more space.
7. Notice what happens.
8. Notice if some part of your body wants to move in a certain way:
   a. Your hand may want to curl into a fist.
   b. Your foot may want to kick.
   c. Your teeth may want to bite.
   d. You may want to shake something.
   e. You may want to punch.
9. Allow your body to make that motion while following the rules listed above. (Following the rules puts boundaries around your body's expression and keeps it healthy for you and others.)
   a. Punch or kick air
   b. Bite a folded napkin or teething ring

       c. Shake or punch a pillow

10. Allow your body full motion while protecting yourself and anyone around you.

11. Allow the motion to shift if it wants to (within the rules):

    a. While your teeth bite a teething ring or folded cloth, you may also want to growl.

    b. While punching the air, you may also want to yell.

    c. While kicking an imaginary behind, you may also want to scream.

    d. Your body may want to go from punching the air to kicking an imaginary behind.

12. Keep allowing the expression of the feeling, as long as that impulse is flowing from your center's focus. Always keep yourself within the rules. Never hurt yourself or anyone else.

13. It may help to imagine the target—someone's face, for example. But, again, let it be a picture in the air that is receiving those punches.

14. You may have an insight about what you want them to feel. For example, as you punch the air, you might realize you want that other person to feel what it's like to be punched in the gut.

15. The particular way this feeling wants to express itself will usually carry great wisdom. As you express the feeling in this manner, you may receive that wisdom, a brilliant insight. For example, you may realize that you

felt punched in the gut when that person was disloyal.

16. This expression will very likely peter out on its own, sooner than you thought it would.

17. The feeling may turn into a different feeling. If it does, make room for the new feeling.

18. It may offer you an insight. You may suddenly realize something.

19. It may—poof—disappear.

20. Notice what is happening in your body right now?

Notice Yourself

How did that go? Was it manageable? How do you feel right now?

Did you get an insight or wisdom about how you were affected by the other person.

You may, if you think it would be helpful, jot down some notes about what you learned from this. Or you can tell a friend.

Most women fear their

> **Facebook**
>
> If you want to talk about your experience on Facebook, remember two things:
>
> 1. It will be there **forever**. Even if you delete it 2 minutes later, it will have flown into thousands of computers. And most future bosses will be able to find it.
> 2. You can, and should, make a deliberate choice about who can view your comments.

anger and tamp it down. They fear that if they let it out, it will never stop. My experience with clients is that they let out a little bit, discover nothing bad happens, and can then let out a little more.

You might want to gather some anger tools. If you tend to want to bite something, a teething ring lets you bite without hurting your teeth. If you like punching, get a big pillow with lots of give. If you want to beat something, get a foam bat and use it against a cushion or your bed.

You can slap water, throw ice, rip paper apart.

The really cool thing is that you don't actually have to hurt anything to get relief, to get through it, or to get insight. It's the muscular motion—the flow of the feeling from inside your body, through your muscles, into the universe—that transforms the feeling.

Whenever a feeling is given this much room and is released safely, you will get something good from it.–4

Space vs. Emptiness

Sometimes people are surprised by the experience of having inner space after Making Room. When you're not used to it, you might mistake it for emptiness. It is not emptiness. It is space.

It is not loneliness. It does not need to be filled. Don't go looking for a different addiction or compulsion. Resist the temptation to fill it up right away. Don't act on that temptation. (Of course you can always make room for the experience of temptation.)

This new space is not emptiness. It is like a womb, a creative chamber. Sit with it. Notice it. See what starts to emerge inside of you.

You'll start to be aware that there is something you've always wanted to learn or to try. Until that comes to you, give yourself positive stimulation. Cultivate a new friendship. Go to a

---

4 Want to work with an expert on these processes? Go to www.systemscentered.com for workshops and consultants.

new or different park. Spend a morning in a museum or art gallery. Peruse a college catalogue. Notice what grabs your eye.

Optional Experiment

Making room can even work on physical pain. We tend to shy away from feeling physical pain. We distract ourselves somehow, trying to be less aware of it. The next time something in your body hurts, pause and give that pain all your attention. Notice what happens.

Practice Practice Practice

The more you practice Making Room, the better you'll get at it.

You will have more energy. You'll learn that your feelings always carry wisdom about your reaction to the world. Once you have this information, you can know more about what you want and what to do.

As you learn to make room, all sorts of other practices will deepen. If you meditate, it will become more profound. If you walk in the woods, you will become more a part of nature. If you create, you will find brilliant new avenues of expression.

If you have a spiritual practice, you will find deeper connection with your Source.

You will have clearer discernment of the actions and motivations of others.

You will carry more authority.

Others will notice and their respect will increase.

You will make choices that are more aligned with your priorities. You will discover new awareness, deeper insights. You will realize you know the direction you should take next.

And, oh yeah, you'll have far less need to eat to cover feelings.[5]

```
SELF RESEARCH
2 Jan.  41 coins
7 Jan.  Change 1a. 31 coins.
12 Jan. Change 1. 23 coins.
19 Jan. Change 2. 19 coins.
26 Jan. Change 3.  12 coins.
```

[5] Want more tools? Get *Your Appetite Switch* by Anne Katherine.

10 Dynorphin, Endorphin, Enkephalin —Oh My

We come now to the most challenging of the changes.

By instituting the first 3 changes, you have helped make Change 4 more manageable. Once Change 4 is more routine, it will support the previous 3 Changes. It's all good.

However, reaching that happy place will take about three weeks of discomfort, disorientation, and irritation.

Are you game?

Remember, after too many years of fighting with your body's chemicals, you are only 3 weeks away from peace. You might put a big red circle on your calendar around the date that is three weeks from now. It will help you remember—when your brain objects to this change—that this unsettling experience is temporary.

And your brain *will* object. We call it withdrawal. That sounds too tame.

You've already learned about 3 chemical processes that make you binge eat:

1. Too much NPY. Too little PYY.

2. Depleted Serotonin.

3. Stress

Next is the big kahuna of the appetite chemicals—internal opiates or opioids.

That's right. Your body can manufacture chemicals that have a structure similar to the kind of opiates that people get seriously addicted to.

And, of course, you can become addicted to those internal opiates as well.

These chemicals are classed as analgesics, painkillers. Yes, just as opiates reduce pain, so do these internal opioids.

The need for pain relief is what, as children, caused us to turn to food. We found something that helped us survive. We were successful.

Now, as adults, we can learn to use safer methods to reduce pain, including setting boundaries around people or situations that cause pain.[6] You've already started. With changes 2 and 3, you began reducing stress, and, therefore, have reduced your need for pain relief.

Internal opiates come in different varieties such as dynophin (major appetite chemical that also may lower body temperature and increase the desire for a high fat diet), beta-endorphin, other endorphins, and enkephalins.

We don't need to identify which internal opiate is controlling us. We just need to know what triggers their release.

---

[6] Found in *Boundaries, Where You End and I Begin* or *Where to Draw the Line*, both by Anne Katherine.

For most people, that trigger is sugar. Many people are also triggered by eating fat. Put sugar and fat together? Zowie!

There's only one surefire way to stop being triggered. Stop eating the trigger. Yep, that's the bad news. The most powerful way to stop being triggered to overeat is to stop eating foods that contain sugar.

Change 4. Abstain from trigger foods, one at a time.

Is it easy at first? No.

Will it get easier? Much.

Are you gonna enjoy this part of the process? No.

Just what do I mean by abstinence? No sugar. No foods containing refined sugar. None. Nada.

Abstinence means to refrain from eating any food containing added sugar. It's a long list, but I'm guessing you are already an expert on ingredients. Just in case:

Refined Sugar Products

Candy	Jam
Sweet baked goods	Sweet bread
Frozen desserts	Syrup
Jelly	Soda/Soft Drinks
Canned Fruit in syrup	

Setting up Success—Preparation for Abstinence

If you truly want to succeed with Change 4, prepare. Do the following things before you start abstinence.

➤ Cleanse your house of all refined sugar foods. (Put all the sugar products in your house in a box. Ask a friend to take the box for a month and after that time, you'll tell her what to do with it.)

- Cleanse your car of all refined sugar foods. Get rid of the wrappers and bags too. The sight of empty wrappers can trigger you, especially when you are first abstinent.
- Cleanse your desk and work area of all refined sugar foods and empty wrappers.
- Tell anyone you live with that you do not want them to eat sugar foods in front of you, and that they will have to dispose of wrappers immediately themselves.
- (If they disregard your request, you will learn something about your relationship.
  - First, make room for your feelings about this.
  - Second, collect the wrappers or partly eaten items and put them in their bed between the sheets—half kidding. Following the rules in the previous chapter, don't hurt them or anything valuable, but it's okay to inconvenience them.)
- Prepare to avoid TV commercials. Set up your TV to record all your shows for 3 weeks. When you watch your programs, fast forward through all the commercials so that you can limit your exposure to visual triggers.
- Prepare to avoid magazine triggers. If you can stand it, plan to not look at your magazines for 3 weeks.
- Do a good shopping.
- Lay in all the snack materials you'll need for at least one week.
  - Buy fruit you really like.
  - Get your tryptophan foods.
  - Get unsweetened soy milk if you like it.
- Don't buy foods or drinks containing sucralose, equal, splenda,

or aspartame. Besides causing harm to your body and, in some cases, making your body resistant to weight loss, they mess up abstinence.

➤ Map your supermarket in your mind. During the first 3 weeks of abstinence, plan to shop only the aisles with fruit, vegetables, meat, and dairy.

➤ Plan to avoid being triggered by smell.

  o The problem with food scents is that they reach the brain sooner than we can think about it. Scent neurons bypass the thinking part of the brain. This means that we could reach for that smelly donut before we know what we are doing. Plan to stay out of bakeries, bakery sections, and stores that deliberately pipe food smells to lure you in.

  o You can go to restaurants during the first 3 weeks, but don't go to one with a tempting bakery display near the front or one that is part bakery.

➤ Plan to avoid making important decisions for at least 3 weeks. Make any decisions with an immediate deadline before you start abstinence.

➤ Decide if you want to be accountable to someone. If so, pick a person you trust, tell them what you are about to do, and ask if you can report to them each day for three weeks. A report would be to email, text, or call them with something like the following message:

  o "I made it through another day. I lost it over a tissue on the floor, and I can't remember why I'm doing this, but I'm proud of making it through 3 days of abstinence."

➤ If they want more details about how to help you, refer them to my book, *Lick It!*, which is for the family and friends of people with appetite disorder.

➤ Decide now how much you want to share on social media. If you want to share on Facebook with just your close friends, choose close friends on your comment pane now, before you start.

The Big Day

Decide on what day you will start, and be careful to get good sleep beforehand. Abstinence is stressful at first. Tryptophan intake will help with that. Be very sure you have stocked your body up on tryptophan by eating your preferred tryptophan foods the day before.

1. Plan to eat fruit at least 3 times a day throughout the 3 weeks. Natural sugars will help you manage the withdrawal.

2. For some of us, soy milk kills cravings. (It has to be unsweetened.)

3. Don't ingest foods or drinks with sucralose, equal, splenda, or aspartame. *Stevia ? Truvia?*

4. Plan some distracting things to do when you get home from work. Like to work puzzles, knit, play the flute? Plan to immerse yourself in your interests after work.

5. Take a walk in a beautiful place. If you normally stop at a comforting restaurant on your way home from work, plan to stop at a soul-nourishing place instead.

6. Pamper yourself with non-food interests. Love the zoo?

Go there. Like movies? Watch them at home. Or if you go to a theatre, ask a friend to get your popcorn for you so you don't have to look at the candy counter. Go to a spa. Have a pedicure. Schedule a massage. You get to have quality non-food treats during this time.

Achieving Abstinence—What to Expect

The first day may not be too bad. It *will* be a change in your routine if you are used to eating sugar at a particular time.

For example, if you plunge into a sugary dessert after you get home from work and if that plunge is the best part of your day, it's gonna feel empty when you get home from work. That's why you prepared in advance to have something different to do when you got home.

Do not plan to do unpleasant things. For example, I've had clients plan to clear out a cluttered room or go through all their magazines or jewelry. **No.** For one thing, you won't always be thinking clearly, and for another, you are already doing something unpleasant. Don't make it worse.

Some people have trouble sleeping for awhile. Some get irritable. Some get unreasonable. Give yourself permission to be a little whacked out. (Don't hurt yourself or anyone else.)

Opioids are painkillers. As they wane, you may feel pain more acutely. Take a safer over-the-counter analgesic for your physical pain. (Don't exceed the recommended dose.)

Remember, an addiction to any type of food is a chemical process. You can only be addicted to something if that substance causes an addictive chain reaction within a certain part of your brain.

This means that the brain will not like it when it no longer gets its chemical. It will be cunning about trying to trick you into eating the food that will restore the missing chemical.

As you hold to your resolve, the brain will have a fit, sort of like a 2 year old having a tantrum at the cash register.

This is why you planned so well ahead of time. You have to find a way to stay on course and not be tricked by your brain.

These first weeks will be disorienting. You are changing your routine, your comfort, and your chemicals all at once. You'll forget what you're doing. You'll forget why you're doing it. This will seem like a stupid and unnecessary idea. You'll convince yourself you aren't addicted.

Of course you wouldn't go through this if you weren't addicted. Withdrawal is nature's way of telling you that you are in fact addicted. [7]

Just in case you get an easy withdrawal, know this. In my experience with hundreds of people getting abstinent, about 10% have *one* easy withdrawal. That causes them to think they aren't addicted and they are prone to losing their abstinence pretty quickly. (But why would they fight abstinence if they weren't addicted?)

Then their next try at abstinence is a bear. Nearly everyone who had an easy withdrawal only had it easy once. From then on,

---

[7] The problem with marijuana is that the withdrawal from pot is so gradual that people can tell themselves they aren't addicted. I mention pot here, because if you use weed recreationally, it triggers eating. You'll have to test for yourself if making the 4 Changes counter-balances the appetite stimulation from pot, or if you want liberation from food struggles enough to let go of that too.

it was very hard to achieve abstinence. So if you are one of the lucky ones, don't throw it away and don't kid yourself.

The first 2 days can be kind of a lark. "Isn't this better than I thought it would be? Anne Katherine exaggerated. I didn't need all that preparation."

For most people, it gets really hard on the 3rd day. And then it gets harder on days 4, 5, and 6. On the 7th day, it gets a little bit easier.

The 2nd week is more manageable.

The 3rd week is more manageable still.

One day, the withdrawal will suddenly lift. The worst will be over. You'll suddenly notice that your thinking is really clear. It is clearer than you can't remember when.

Congratulations!

And you aren't done. Just like the first 3 Changes, the 4th Change must be maintained.

When the worst is over, your addicted brain may tell you you never were addicted and all this abstinence is unnecessary. It may even lie. It may say, "Ah, withdrawal wasn't that bad." It is conveniently forgetting that you wanted to throw a chair through the window, yell at your sister, and eat a bakery.

Thoughts like that are typical for addicted people. The addicted brain is cunning but not smart about addiction. It will still try to pull you back into "using" sugar.

It will have certain times that it will exert extra pressure to get you to fall off the wagon. The usual times of extra pressure are after 3 months, 6 months, and 9 months of abstinence. Ditto every anniversary of achieving abstinence for about 5 years.

This is why addicts celebrate their abstinence birthdays.

It's a big deal, a great big achievement to stay abstinent, and it's important to remember that the brain will still try to get you back to the addiction even years into abstinence.

Your brain will also crave sugar any time stress increases in your life, or when something really difficult happens.

Support. An abstinent friend can be a giant help at these times. You can also find free support at Overeaters Anonymous and Food Addicts Anonymous. All 12 step programs—AA, NA, etc.—have experts on recovery who will offer support. These people understand the power of addiction and they know how to listen and talk about it in a way that maintains abstinence.

Journaling. Many find it useful to journal, to record their feelings and thoughts, especially during the first 3 weeks of abstinence. Then they have a record to refer to if the addicted brain tells them it wasn't too bad.

FAQ

Q. I'm just as addicted to bread as to sugar. Should I get abstinent from both at the same time?

A. If and only if you are in an effective support group with other abstinent people. For example, FAA does promote a wider abstinence all at once. If you are using this support and the group is dependable, try it. But if most of the people in the group have not had success with long term abstinence, they can give you emotional support, but have themselves bitten off more than they can chew.

Q. After I'm abstinent from sugar, do I have to get abstinent from fatty foods?

A. You should never get abstinent from all foods with oil and fat, because you need certain nutrients that are only carried in such foods. You can get abstinent from certain types of fatty foods, or you can set a limit. For example, you could get abstinent from fried foods or limit your intake to one fried food per week.

Q. After I'm abstinent from sugar, should I get abstinent from breads and other refined starches?

A. You must not add to your abstinence until you've had a good solid abstinence from sugar for one year, unless you have support from people who have long term abstinence. If, and only if, you are in an effective 12 step program or in a group with lots of dependable support, should you try to expand your abstinence. If you do this too soon with not enough support, you will sabotage your sugar abstinence and be back face down in the crumbs.

Q. If I can set a limit for fat, why can't I set a similar limit for sugar?

A. Think of sugar as being an addiction similar to cigarettes. Very, very few people can smoke one cigarette a day after being addicted to nicotine. After people quit smoking, they usually try to test this by smoking just one cigarette. Zoom. They are smoking full tilt right away.

Same thing with alcoholics. Once people are sober, they must refrain from all alcohol. One sip could torpedo their sobriety, even if that sip occurs 10 years after their first abstinence. This is why we celebrate sobriety birthdays. Making it another year is a big deal. The mechanism in the brain for alcoholism is almost identical to the mechanism for food addiction. And this mechanism doesn't go away, even when it's inactive.

Q. I'm actually more addicted to fat than sugar. I don't eat that many sweets.

A. But are the fatty foods you eat also sweet? If so, it's still a better idea to start with sugar. Sugar abstinence is a challenge to achieve, but moderation with fat is even harder, and since you have to continue to eat fat, the boundary is less clear. At least with sugar abstinence you have a clear boundary—none. No refined sugar. If the fat foods you crave are not sweet or contain no sugar, you can start by eliminating all fried foods, but pay close attention.

If your starch and/or sugar intake goes up, your brain is substituting another substance to handle withdrawal. If this happens, start over, with sugar abstinence. After that is firmly established—at least 6 months—then eliminate battered foods that are cooked in hot oil like fried chicken, fish, and onion rings.

It's a Cat Nap

Maintain your abstinence. It is far easier to maintain abstinence than to regain it.

On the other hand, relapse is a common part of addiction. Eventually we want to test whether we are still addicted to our most coveted substance, and then we relapse. The brain *roars* out of its nap and *wants* its stuff.

Really? You might say. After going to all that trouble, I would risk losing abstinence? Yep. Happens every day. The brain has an endless supply of excuses for using again. With my own clients, the most dangerous sentence they ever said was, "I know I'll never eat sugar again."

What's wrong with this positive thinking?

It's ignoring the power of addiction. It's testifying that we think we're in control of the addiction, that we can control the addiction.

We can't. We can't control an addiction. When it is activated, it controls us.

We can surrender to the reality, to the knowledge that the addictive chain reaction is inside us all the time, that it looks for its chance to get back on top, that it will use anything, that it has no principles.

When we stay clear about that reality, we know we have to create the environment that puts the addiction to sleep. We have to be abstinent, and we have to maintain our satiety chemicals. We also have to protect ourselves from being too hungry, too angry, too lonely, or too tired. We stay clear about the fact that our brains will use any trick to break our resolve.

The addicted part of the brain may go to sleep during abstinence, but it is just a nap—with a defective snooze button.

One Day at a Time

When you achieve abstinence, you will have made Change 4. Remember to maintain all 4 changes, today. Today. And today.

It's that One Day at a Time thing. Keep it manageable. You only have to maintain the 4 changes today.

Tomorrow, it will be today. Tomorrow, maintain the changes for today.

Post-Test

After you've beaten withdrawal and all 4 Changes are on, do your self research at least one more time. This will give an independent sort of proof, beyond your own feelings (which could be hard to remember later) that the 4 Changes really did change your relationship with food and eating.

I had a beloved client who was so self-critical that she was sure that her brain had not cooperated even after making these changes.

I had to pull out her charts and show her the drastic drop in food involvement before she could even begin to entertain the idea that she might have succeeded at something.

We get into habits of thought, ways of thinking about ourselves, that may not serve us. And may not be accurate. If this could be your story, give yourself actual numbers that show your body's response to your efforts.

SELF RESEARCH
2 Jan. 41 coins
7 Jan. Change 1a. 31 coins.
12 Jan. Change 1. 23 coins.
19 Jan. Change 2. 19 coins.
26 Jan. Change 3. 12 coins.

26 Feb. Change 4. 5 coins.

---

11 What If?

What if you start the first 2 changes, they work, and then you abandon the whole thing?

What if you are rolling along with Changes 1, 2, and 3, and then can't manage Change 4? Will you throw the whole thing out or sustain the first three Changes and tackle Change 4 later?

What if you are wildly successful, you make all 4 Changes, they work, and they make a difference to your eating and appetite? And then one day, you throw out the whole regimen?

Any of the above scenarios give you an important message.

Potential Message 1: You may have a deep, long-standing pattern of self-sabotage that hijacks your success over and over.

If so, the answer is MAA or SSA, Misery Addicts Anonymous or Self-Sabotagers Anonymous. This is a single organization which has evolved in its understanding, hence the two names. The website address is at the end of this book.

You could also get the book, *When Misery is Company*, which gives lots of tools, explanations, and processes for recovery.

Potential Message 2: Something went wrong in your life and you automatically reached for traditional comfort. It happened before you even thought about it.

Review Change 3, go through one of the steps, and get back to your effective routine.

It may also help to talk to someone to remind yourself that human comfort can actually be more soothing.

Potential Message 3: You don't have enough support. These changes are turning out to ask more of you than you can sustain on your own. Talking to someone will help you discover what issue is being triggered—either because the changes made your mind clearer or because taking care of yourself feels like you're breaking a rule.

Are you curious about this? Would you like to discover what gets in your way from taking hold of your life in a more productive way?

Talk to somebody you trust.

Potential Message 4: Someone may be actively sabotaging you. Someone may not like you being good to yourself and may have upped demands on you so that you would be too busy or too distracted to attend to the routine that sustains the changes.

If this is happening, it means you became clearer, perhaps were doing a better job staying on course with your own life, and someone didn't like that and wanted you back in attendance on him/her.

If this is the case, insist that the other person read *Lick It! Fix Her Appetite Switch*.

You have a big decision to make:

- Do you want to live for someone else?
- Do you want to live for yourself?

If you choose to make your own life your priority, you may need to have a serious conversation with that person and set a clear boundary. Some examples of boundary-setting statements:

"Because I realize I have to follow a certain routine to be healthier, I will be eating 5 meals and snacks a day. I will take 20 minutes mid-morning and mid-afternoon to do this. Those 20 minutes are mine and I won't be available to you at those times. You will have to take care of yourself."

"When I prepare snacks for myself, I will put them in this red container. This is my food. If you want a snack, you can have anything on this other shelf. My food is off limits."

"On our trip, I will not be eating at that bakery/restaurant we traditionally stop at. You can go. I won't. I will eat at the café around the corner and then we can join each other again afterwards to go to that flea market."

"I am preventing diabetes so I will no longer be eating any food with sugar in it. I will also not cook sweet foods anymore. This shelf has my food. Please do not put any sugary foods on that shelf."

"I choose to not eat sugar. Please do all your sugar eating out of the house/in the basement/in your man cave/before you get home. Please throw away your sugar wrappers, bags, and containers. Are you willing to help me in this way?"

"I want to know if you are willing to support me. Please tell me the truth. Will you respect the limits I need to set for myself?"

What can you do if the other person says they will support

you, but their actions don't back up their words? For more advanced issues, my book *Where to Draw the Line* has many examples of boundaries, including how to make boundaries stronger if they are violated.

The short version is this: if your boundary is not respected, make it stronger, make it more inclusive, and create consequences. Think about what the other person is trying to get from you by defying your limit. You can either give that to them and see if they calm down, or give it to them only when they respect your boundary.

For example, my spouse kept putting knives in the dishpan. I couldn't see them under the water, and eventually got cut. This is after requesting (about 10 times) (Okay, 20 times) that knives not be put in the dishpan. Anger is a consequence and I expressed anger appropriately and directly.

I know my spouse does not want to hurt me and just forgets, but I am unwilling to risk being cut just because there's a benign reason for the lapse.

I set a new boundary. "When I find a knife, I will immediately stop doing the dishes and I won't do them again for ____ days. I will add another day of not doing dishes every time I find a knife in the pan."

This worked. Consequences help a person remember and also motivate them to make a change themselves.

12 Fixing Your Life

Is it over-reaching to say that fixing your over-active appetite will fix your life?

I think not.

When you are constantly fighting the pressure exerted by appetite chemicals, your time and energy are side-tracked from what matters more.

That fight causes you to miss a lot. You might be missing opportunities, gifts, signposts, serendipitous offerings, positive gestures from good people, or possibilities.

We don't know what we are missing. Obviously.

However, when we make these changes, the struggle diminishes and our thinking gets clearer. We suddenly notice good things around us. We notice opportunities. We realize a signpost is right in front of us. We discover a good friendship is available if we'll just show up.

A lot is waiting for you, beyond the food.

I want you to know how important your life is.

I don't say this just out of a philosophical belief.

I *know* this because I've worked with, directly or indirectly, hundreds of people, mostly women, with over-active appetite.

Nearly all of them were sensitive people. That's why they

needed food in the first place.

They were vulnerable to being hurt, they *were* hurt, and they found relief in food.

They were easily hurt because they had a sensitivity to the feelings of others, to the meanness of others, to the needs or desperations of others. The bad actions of other people affected them deeply—because they were sensitive to harsh actions or words and could be affected.

(And other siblings in the same house may not have been harmed so deeply if they were less sensitive or less vulnerable due to more innate protection or shielding. A difference in sibling response to trauma does not alter the reality that trauma existed.)

Nearly all sensitive people have a gift. Many sensitive people put the needs of others before their own needs. Therefore they either don't discover their gift or they don't make time to develop it.

You can now reverse that trend. You can discover and develop your gift.

All you have to do is maintain the 4 Changes.

Remember, you can't set it and forget it. You have to continue to prepare for and deliberately do all 4 Changes. You have to replace those snacks, fill baggies, buy cheese sticks, stick a bag of almonds in your pack. You have to buy that turkey or milk or tahini. You have to Make Room. You have to stay out of slippery places—that is, any place that broadcasts the foods that trigger your appetite or addictive chemicals.

Whenever your appetite starts tuning up, you have an indicator that something has slipped. Either you've gotten less deliberate about your snacks, your tryptophan tank is low, a feeling is being ignored, or you've been playing with the edges of your abstinence.

Look at what needs attention, beef it up (turkey it up?), and watch your appetite chemicals go back to sleep.

Additional Help

Human contact. Good people, who can listen and support you, will help you stay on track. If you want to put together a 4 Changes support group, you'll find Guidelines toward the end of this book.

A spiritual practice. When you open yourself to your Source and make time and space for your Source to refill you, it will always help.

You matter so very much to many of us.

Now, show yourself that you matter to you.

Additional Information

Want the science behind these four changes?

Anne Katherine has other books that illustrate the chemistry behind overeating, food addiction, and the umbrella addiction—addiction to misery or self-sabotage.

Your Appetite Switch

This book includes more details and illustrations of the brain chemistry behind appetite disorder, spaces out the steps, and offers additional tools. The print book has detailed charts that you can use to research your own chemical interactions. Some people are helped by these charts. Others are overwhelmed. It's perfectly okay to read the book and not do any of the charting.

Anatomy of a Food Addiction

This book gives you details on the physiology of an addiction to food, the many similarities to alcoholism, and step-by-step guidance for recovery.

Lick It!

For the family, friends, and helping professionals of people with over-active appetite, especially for those who genuinely want to understand and support you. It shows the brain chemistry of appetite disorder in colorful illustrations and even gives family members a way to vent their own irritation with this dysfunction.

(If they've tried hard to be "nice" and understanding, they

may have anger about the impact of appetite disorder on the family. That anger will leak out in unhelpful ways, so this book gives healthy ways to channel it.)

Some family members scapegoat the person with over-active appetite or blame the person for having it. Families relinquish their scapegoats reluctantly. If you have been a scapegoat, my books on Boundaries will help.

When Misery is Company

If you know what to do to feel better, and can't make yourself do it, if feeling better is scarier than feeling miserable, or if you sabotage yourself over and over, this book describes the umbrella addiction, the one that has people going from one addiction to another, like changing seats on the Titanic. It gives step-by-step methods to stop your own self-sabotage.

Other books to improve your life and put right your relationships and your communities:

Boundaries, Where You End and I Begin

Boundaries bring order to our lives, strengthen our relationships with others and ourselves, and are essential to our mental and physical health. For those of us who have walked away from a conversation, meeting, or visit feeling violated and not understanding why, this book helps us recognize and set healthy boundaries. Real-life stories illustrate the ill effects of not setting limits and the benefits gained by respecting our own boundaries and those of others.

Where to Draw the Line

With every encounter, we either demonstrate that we'll protect what we value or that we'll give ourselves away. Healthy boundaries preserve our integrity. Unlike defenses, which isolate us from our true selves and from those we love, boundaries filter out harm.

This book provides the tools and insights needed to create boundaries so that we can ensure time and energy for the things that matter—and helps break down limiting defenses that stunt personal growth. Focusing on every facet of daily life—from friendships and sexual relationships to dress and appearance to money, food, and psychotherapy—Anne Katherine presents case studies that highlight the ways in which individuals violate their own boundaries or let other people breach them. Using real-life examples, from self-sacrificing mothers to obsessive neat freaks, she offers specific advice on making choices that balance one's own needs with the needs of others.

Boundaries are the unseen structures that support healthy, productive lives. *Where to Draw the Line* shows readers how to strengthen them and hold them in place every day.

Boundaries in an Overconnected World

Are you glued to your devices? Do you know what you are missing? Electronic devices are efficient and save time, but they can steal more than give if they take too much of your attention. Learn how to set limits that protect the quality of your life for yourself and the people who matter to you. Restore human contact to your life and strengthen not just your thumbs but your heart.

The Splintered Cross

Heal, and even make stronger, your spiritual community. Use conflicts to gain powerful new skills that transform, not just the individuals involved, but that strengthen families and are a testimony to others about how to embrace differences and include those who have traditionally been marginalized.

4 Changes Group Guidelines

Support usually helps. Informed, effective support always helps.

Create a 4 Changes support group so that you and your friends can assist each other through this transition in your life. This truly can be a significant turning point for you. It's worth giving yourself every advantage.

Sample Agenda

Centering. A member leads the group in a Prep Step from Chapter 9.

Successes. Going around the circle, everyone shares some achievement. It does not have to be gigantic. It can be an increase in awareness, an insight, a result of Self Research, a noticed difference in appetite, an improvement in self care or eating choices, improved self honesty.

Group Reading. Each week, pick a chapter from this book. Pass the book around the circle. Each member reads one paragraph. Once this book has been read, move on to books on recovery from AA, OA, or other books by Anne Katherine.

Ooops! Or How Old Patterns Tripped Me Up. Going around the circle, members share briefly about a slip or mistake and, if possible, the thought or feeling that led to the old behavior.

Gearing Up. Each member chooses a Change to focus on, start, or improve for the next week.

Advice Wanted. Members that need ideas request help

for **after** the meeting closes. Since giving advice is a lot more fun than focusing on ourselves, only make the ***request*** during the meeting. Actually give and receive advice after Closing.

Closing. A group prayer or affirmation.

Guidelines

- Keep time boundaries. Start and end on time.
- Agree to be both anonymous and confidential.
  - *Anonymous* means you protect the identity of other members by not revealing their names or characteristics that would identify them to people outside the meeting.
  - *Confidential* means you protect the content of what people share about themselves. Don't pass on stories or comments made by others.
- Agree that you will refrain from giving advice or suggestions until after the Closing. We are easily distracted into making someone a project and it is much simpler to fix others than to fix ourselves.
- Do not socialize within the meeting.
- After each person shares, say thank you or clap. Then move on.
- Do not cross talk.
  - Cross talk means jumping in with a response to someone's comment. The goal is for you to use the meeting to focus on your own internal process. If you aren't distracted into "helping," you can 'work along' while someone else talks.

- o   When cross talk is allowed, everyone downstream from that person will get less time. Therefore, keep the discipline of listening respectfully to each person's share and moving on.
- Be brief in your sharing. Each person will get at least 3 chances to talk if everyone keeps the meeting moving.
- Notice if time is being used up by someone who indulges in long explanations. They may be entertaining, but what is that costing members who get less time as a result?

Personal Sharing—Making a distinction

Our sharing at a support meeting—or actually communication in a variety of places that have the potential to be meaningful (church, in therapy, with an intimate)—can take two different forms.

- Exploration
- Explanation

We can talk to explore or to explain.

Exploring is enormously productive. Our words may be hesitant, we may pause often, because we are looking inside as we talk. We are exploring our inner landscape and we are discovering new awareness as we talk.

Explaining means we are telling a story of which we already know the end. Explaining uses up time and doesn't get us anywhere new. We are relating what we already know and keeping ourselves from discovering something new.   This type of talk is quicker, it uses our common catch phrases, it may have a certain singsong tone.